Workout Log Book

DETAILS

NAME

ADDRESS

E-MAIL ADDRESS

WEBSITE

PHONE **FAX**

EMERGENCY CONTACT PERSON

PHONE **FAX**

LOG BOOK DETAILS

CONTINUED FROM LOG BOOK

LOG START DATE

CONTINUED TO LOG BOOK

LOG END DATE

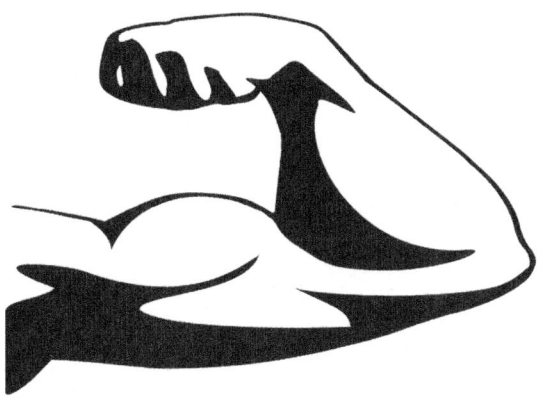

"Definition of a really good workout: when you hate doing it, but you love finishing it."

Enjoying this Book?

Please leave a review because we would love to hear your feedback, opinions, and advice to create better products and services for you! Also, We want to know how you creatively use your Logbook and Planner.

Thank you for your support.
You are greatly appreciated!

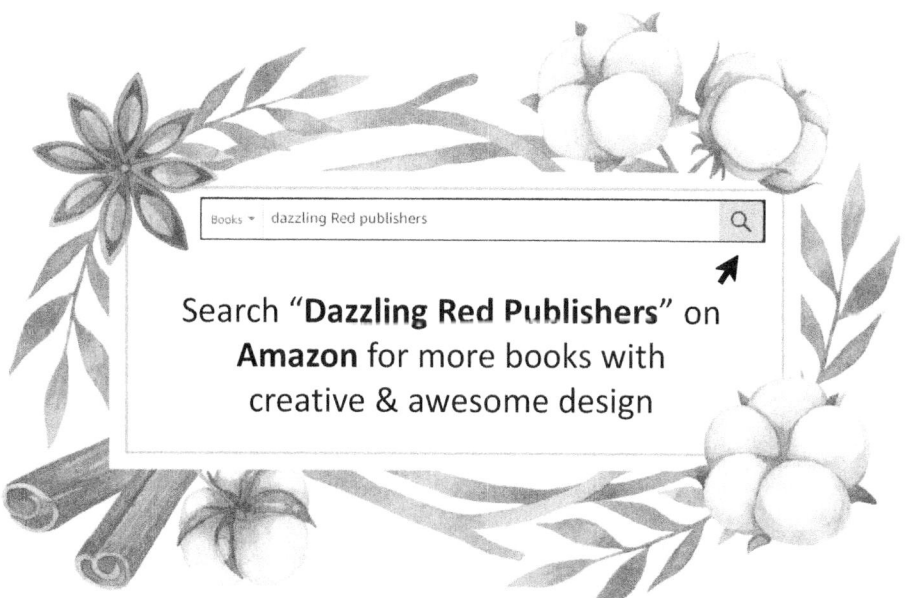

Search **"Dazzling Red Publishers"** on **Amazon** for more books with creative & awesome design

Dazzling Publishers

Copyright © 2020 all Rights Reserved

Workout Log Book

Date ....

WEIGHT　　　　　　MON / TUE / WED / THU / FRI / SAT / SUN

MUSCLE GROUP　　　HOW I FEEL　　1 / 2 / 3 / 4 / 5 / 6

START TIME　　　　　FINISH TIME

WATER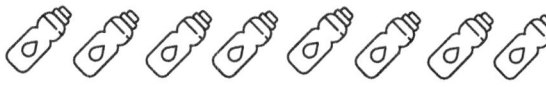

STRENGTH TRAINING

☐ UPPER BODY　　☐ LOWER BODY　　☐ ABS

CARDIO

EXERCISE	TIME	DISTANCE	CALS BURNED

EXERCISE	SET	1	2	3	4	5	6
	REPS						
	WEIGHT						
	REPS						
	WEIGHT						
	REPS						
	WEIGHT						
	REPS						
	WEIGHT						
	REPS						
	WEIGHT						
	REPS						
	WEIGHT						

EXERCISE	SET	1	2	3	4	5	6
	REPS						
	WEIGHT						
	REPS						
	WEIGHT						
	REPS						
	WEIGHT						
	REPS						
	WEIGHT						
	REPS						
	WEIGHT						
	REPS						
	WEIGHT						

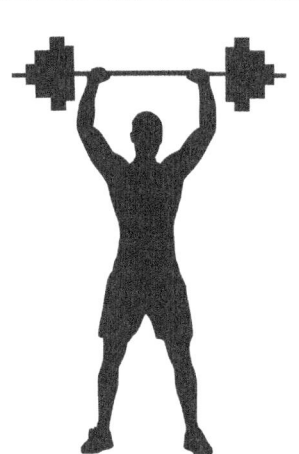

MEASUREMENTS	
NECK	
R BICEP	
L BICEP	
CHEST	
WAIST	
HIPS	
R THIGH	
L THIGH	
CALF	

NOTES

....
....
....
....
....
....
....
....
....
....
....

Workout Log Book

Date ....

WEIGHT MON / TUE / WED / THU / FRI / SAT / SUN

MUSCLE GROUP HOW I FEEL 1 / 2 / 3 / 4 / 5 / 6

START TIME FINISH TIME

WATER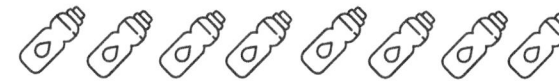

STRENGTH TRAINING

☐ UPPER BODY ☐ LOWER BODY ☐ ABS

CARDIO

EXERCISE	TIME	DISTANCE	CALS BURNED

EXERCISE	SET	1	2	3	4	5	6
	REPS						
	WEIGHT						
	REPS						
	WEIGHT						
	REPS						
	WEIGHT						
	REPS						
	WEIGHT						
	REPS						
	WEIGHT						
	REPS						
	WEIGHT						

EXERCISE	SET	1	2	3	4	5	6
	REPS						
	WEIGHT						
	REPS						
	WEIGHT						
	REPS						
	WEIGHT						
	REPS						
	WEIGHT						
	REPS						
	WEIGHT						
	REPS						
	WEIGHT						

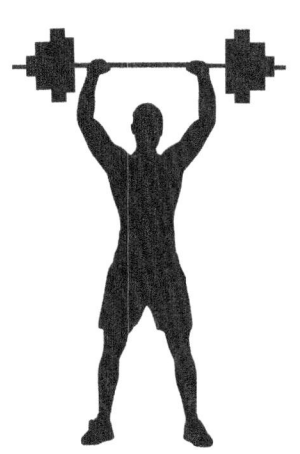

MEASUREMENTS	
NECK	
R BICEP	
L BICEP	
CHEST	
WAIST	
HIPS	
R THIGH	
L THIGH	
CALF	

NOTES

....
....
....
....
....
....
....
....
....
....
....

Workout Log Book

Date ....

WEIGHT　　　　　　MON / TUE / WED / THU / FRI / SAT / SUN

MUSCLE GROUP　　　HOW I FEEL　 1 / 2 / 3 / 4 / 5 / 6

START TIME　　　　　FINISH TIME

WATER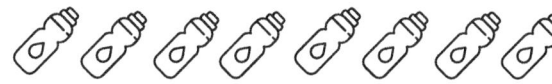

STRENGTH TRAINING

☐ UPPER BODY　　☐ LOWER BODY　　☐ ABS

CARDIO

EXERCISE	TIME	DISTANCE	CALS BURNED

EXERCISE	SET	1	2	3	4	5	6
	REPS						
	WEIGHT						
	REPS						
	WEIGHT						
	REPS						
	WEIGHT						
	REPS						
	WEIGHT						
	REPS						
	WEIGHT						
	REPS						
	WEIGHT						

EXERCISE	SET	1	2	3	4	5	6
	REPS						
	WEIGHT						
	REPS						
	WEIGHT						
	REPS						
	WEIGHT						
	REPS						
	WEIGHT						
	REPS						
	WEIGHT						
	REPS						
	WEIGHT						

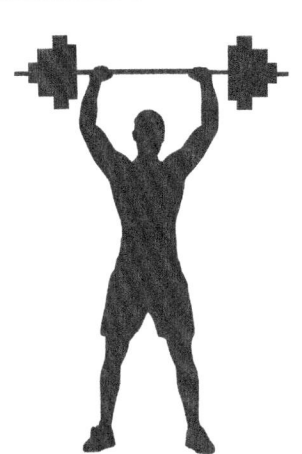

MEASUREMENTS	
NECK	
R BICEP	
L BICEP	
CHEST	
WAIST	
HIPS	
R THIGH	
L THIGH	
CALF	

NOTES

....
....
....
....
....
....
....
....
....
....

Workout Log Book

Date ....

WEIGHT　　　　　　　MON / TUE / WED / THU / FRI / SAT / SUN

MUSCLE GROUP　　　　HOW I FEEL　1 / 2 / 3 / 4 / 5 / 6

START TIME　　　　　 FINISH TIME

WATER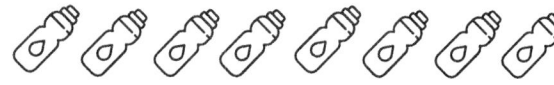

STRENGTH TRAINING

☐ UPPER BODY　　☐ LOWER BODY　　☐ ABS

CARDIO

EXERCISE	TIME	DISTANCE	CALS BURNED

EXERCISE	SET	1	2	3	4	5	6
	REPS						
	WEIGHT						
	REPS						
	WEIGHT						
	REPS						
	WEIGHT						
	REPS						
	WEIGHT						
	REPS						
	WEIGHT						
	REPS						
	WEIGHT						

EXERCISE	SET	1	2	3	4	5	6
	REPS						
	WEIGHT						
	REPS						
	WEIGHT						
	REPS						
	WEIGHT						
	REPS						
	WEIGHT						
	REPS						
	WEIGHT						
	REPS						
	WEIGHT						

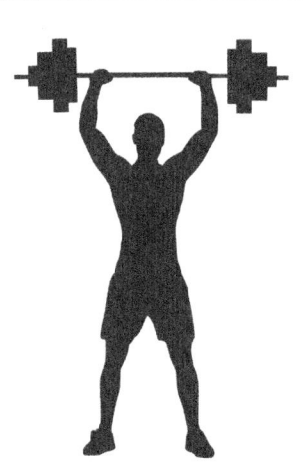

MEASUREMENTS	
NECK	
R BICEP	
L BICEP	
CHEST	
WAIST	
HIPS	
R THIGH	
L THIGH	
CALF	

NOTES

....
....
....
....
....
....
....
....
....
....

Workout Log Book

Date ....

WEIGHT

MUSCLE GROUP

START TIME

MON / TUE / WED / THU / FRI / SAT / SUN

HOW I FEEL   1 / 2 / 3 / 4 / 5 / 6

FINISH TIME

WATER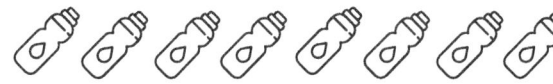

STRENGTH TRAINING

☐ UPPER BODY   ☐ LOWER BODY   ☐ ABS

CARDIO

EXERCISE	TIME	DISTANCE	CALS BURNED

EXERCISE	SET	1	2	3	4	5	6
	REPS						
	WEIGHT						
	REPS						
	WEIGHT						
	REPS						
	WEIGHT						
	REPS						
	WEIGHT						
	REPS						
	WEIGHT						
	REPS						
	WEIGHT						

EXERCISE	SET	1	2	3	4	5	6
	REPS						
	WEIGHT						
	REPS						
	WEIGHT						
	REPS						
	WEIGHT						
	REPS						
	WEIGHT						
	REPS						
	WEIGHT						
	REPS						
	WEIGHT						

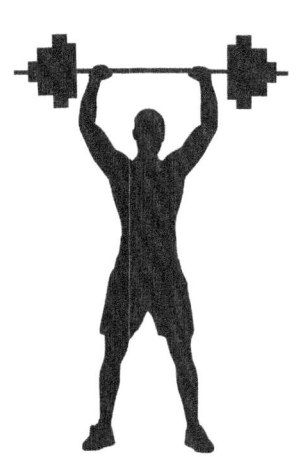

MEASUREMENTS	
NECK	
R BICEP	
L BICEP	
CHEST	
WAIST	
HIPS	
R THIGH	
L THIGH	
CALF	

NOTES

....
....
....
....
....
....
....
....
....
....
....

Workout Log Book

Date ....

WEIGHT MON / TUE / WED / THU / FRI / SAT / SUN

MUSCLE GROUP HOW I FEEL 1 / 2 / 3 / 4 / 5 / 6

START TIME FINISH TIME

WATER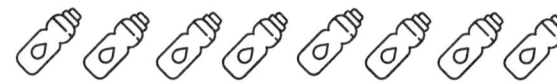

STRENGTH TRAINING

☐ UPPER BODY ☐ LOWER BODY ☐ ABS

CARDIO

EXERCISE	TIME	DISTANCE	CALS BURNED

EXERCISE	SET	1	2	3	4	5	6
	REPS						
	WEIGHT						
	REPS						
	WEIGHT						
	REPS						
	WEIGHT						
	REPS						
	WEIGHT						
	REPS						
	WEIGHT						
	REPS						
	WEIGHT						

EXERCISE	SET	1	2	3	4	5	6
	REPS						
	WEIGHT						
	REPS						
	WEIGHT						
	REPS						
	WEIGHT						
	REPS						
	WEIGHT						
	REPS						
	WEIGHT						
	REPS						
	WEIGHT						

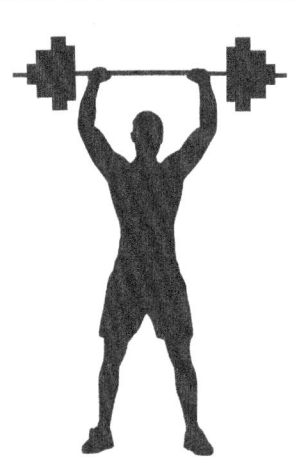

MEASUREMENTS	
NECK	
R BICEP	
L BICEP	
CHEST	
WAIST	
HIPS	
R THIGH	
L THIGH	
CALF	

NOTES

....
....
....
....
....
....
....
....
....
....

Workout Log Book

Date ....

WEIGHT MON / TUE / WED / THU / FRI / SAT / SUN

MUSCLE GROUP HOW I FEEL 1 / 2 / 3 / 4 / 5 / 6

START TIME FINISH TIME

WATER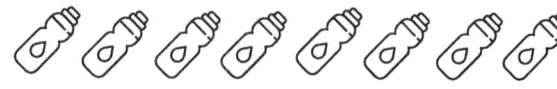

STRENGTH TRAINING

☐ UPPER BODY   ☐ LOWER BODY   ☐ ABS

CARDIO

EXERCISE	TIME	DISTANCE	CALS BURNED

EXERCISE	SET	1	2	3	4	5	6
	REPS						
	WEIGHT						
	REPS						
	WEIGHT						
	REPS						
	WEIGHT						
	REPS						
	WEIGHT						
	REPS						
	WEIGHT						
	REPS						
	WEIGHT						

EXERCISE	SET	1	2	3	4	5	6
	REPS						
	WEIGHT						
	REPS						
	WEIGHT						
	REPS						
	WEIGHT						
	REPS						
	WEIGHT						
	REPS						
	WEIGHT						
	REPS						
	WEIGHT						

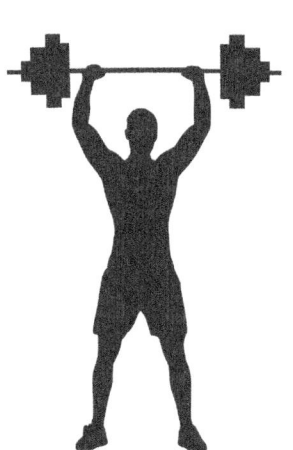

MEASUREMENTS	
NECK	
R BICEP	
L BICEP	
CHEST	
WAIST	
HIPS	
R THIGH	
L THIGH	
CALF	

NOTES

....
....
....
....
....
....
....
....
....
....
....

Workout Log Book

Date ....

WEIGHT

MUSCLE GROUP

START TIME

MON / TUE / WED / THU / FRI / SAT / SUN

HOW I FEEL   1 / 2 / 3 / 4 / 5 / 6

FINISH TIME

WATER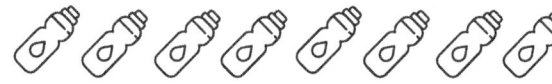

STRENGTH TRAINING

☐ UPPER BODY   ☐ LOWER BODY   ☐ ABS

CARDIO

EXERCISE	TIME	DISTANCE	CALS BURNED

EXERCISE	SET	1	2	3	4	5	6
	REPS						
	WEIGHT						
	REPS						
	WEIGHT						
	REPS						
	WEIGHT						
	REPS						
	WEIGHT						
	REPS						
	WEIGHT						
	REPS						
	WEIGHT						

EXERCISE	SET	1	2	3	4	5	6
	REPS						
	WEIGHT						
	REPS						
	WEIGHT						
	REPS						
	WEIGHT						
	REPS						
	WEIGHT						
	REPS						
	WEIGHT						
	REPS						
	WEIGHT						

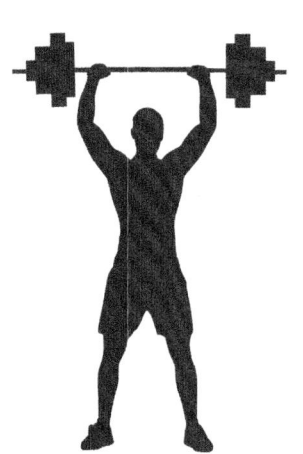

MEASUREMENTS	
NECK	
R BICEP	
L BICEP	
CHEST	
WAIST	
HIPS	
R THIGH	
L THIGH	
CALF	

NOTES

....
....
....
....
....
....
....
....
....
....

Workout Log Book

Date ....

WEIGHT　　　　　　MON / TUE / WED / THU / FRI / SAT / SUN

MUSCLE GROUP　　　HOW I FEEL　　1 / 2 / 3 / 4 / 5 / 6

START TIME　　　　　FINISH TIME

WATER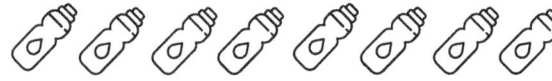

STRENGTH TRAINING

☐ UPPER BODY　　☐ LOWER BODY　　☐ ABS

CARDIO

EXERCISE	TIME	DISTANCE	CALS BURNED

EXERCISE	SET	1	2	3	4	5	6
	REPS						
	WEIGHT						
	REPS						
	WEIGHT						
	REPS						
	WEIGHT						
	REPS						
	WEIGHT						
	REPS						
	WEIGHT						
	REPS						
	WEIGHT						

EXERCISE	SET	1	2	3	4	5	6
	REPS						
	WEIGHT						
	REPS						
	WEIGHT						
	REPS						
	WEIGHT						
	REPS						
	WEIGHT						
	REPS						
	WEIGHT						
	REPS						
	WEIGHT						

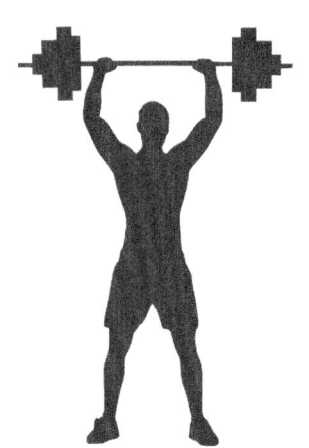

MEASUREMENTS	
NECK	
R BICEP	
L BICEP	
CHEST	
WAIST	
HIPS	
R THIGH	
L THIGH	
CALF	

NOTES

....
....
....
....
....
....
....
....
....
....

Workout Log Book

Date ....

WEIGHT　　　　　　　MON / TUE / WED / THU / FRI / SAT / SUN

MUSCLE GROUP　　　HOW I FEEL　　1 / 2 / 3 / 4 / 5 / 6

START TIME　　　　　FINISH TIME

WATER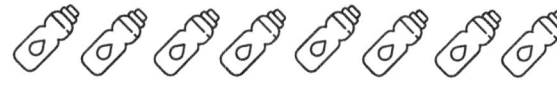

STRENGTH TRAINING

☐ UPPER BODY　　☐ LOWER BODY　　☐ ABS

CARDIO

EXERCISE	TIME	DISTANCE	CALS BURNED

EXERCISE	SET	1	2	3	4	5	6
	REPS						
	WEIGHT						
	REPS						
	WEIGHT						
	REPS						
	WEIGHT						
	REPS						
	WEIGHT						
	REPS						
	WEIGHT						
	REPS						
	WEIGHT						

EXERCISE	SET	1	2	3	4	5	6
	REPS						
	WEIGHT						
	REPS						
	WEIGHT						
	REPS						
	WEIGHT						
	REPS						
	WEIGHT						
	REPS						
	WEIGHT						
	REPS						
	WEIGHT						

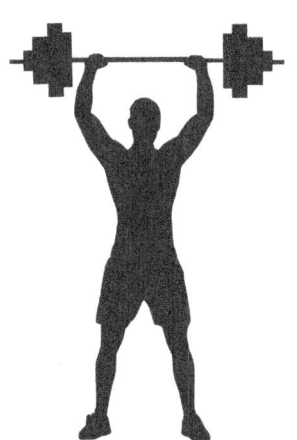

MEASUREMENTS	
NECK	
R BICEP	
L BICEP	
CHEST	
WAIST	
HIPS	
R THIGH	
L THIGH	
CALF	

NOTES

....
....
....
....
....
....
....
....
....
....
....

Workout Log Book

Date ....

WEIGHT MON / TUE / WED / THU / FRI / SAT / SUN

MUSCLE GROUP HOW I FEEL 1 / 2 / 3 / 4 / 5 / 6

START TIME FINISH TIME

WATER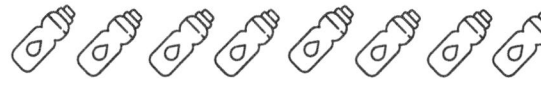

STRENGTH TRAINING

☐ UPPER BODY   ☐ LOWER BODY   ☐ ABS

CARDIO

EXERCISE	TIME	DISTANCE	CALS BURNED

EXERCISE	SET	1	2	3	4	5	6
	REPS						
	WEIGHT						
	REPS						
	WEIGHT						
	REPS						
	WEIGHT						
	REPS						
	WEIGHT						
	REPS						
	WEIGHT						
	REPS						
	WEIGHT						

EXERCISE	SET	1	2	3	4	5	6
	REPS						
	WEIGHT						
	REPS						
	WEIGHT						
	REPS						
	WEIGHT						
	REPS						
	WEIGHT						
	REPS						
	WEIGHT						
	REPS						
	WEIGHT						

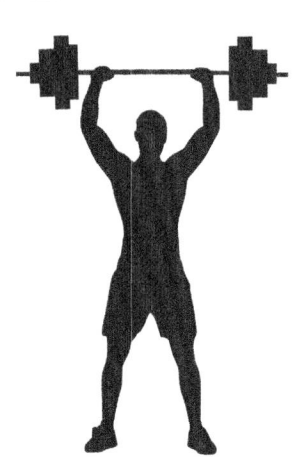

MEASUREMENTS	
NECK	
R BICEP	
L BICEP	
CHEST	
WAIST	
HIPS	
R THIGH	
L THIGH	
CALF	

NOTES

....
....
....
....
....
....
....
....
....
....

Workout Log Book

Date ....

WEIGHT MON / TUE / WED / THU / FRI / SAT / SUN

MUSCLE GROUP HOW I FEEL 1 / 2 / 3 / 4 / 5 / 6

START TIME FINISH TIME

WATER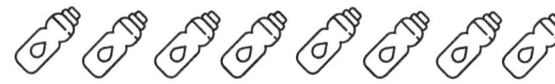

STRENGTH TRAINING

☐ UPPER BODY ☐ LOWER BODY ☐ ABS

CARDIO

EXERCISE	TIME	DISTANCE	CALS BURNED

EXERCISE	SET	1	2	3	4	5	6
	REPS						
	WEIGHT						
	REPS						
	WEIGHT						
	REPS						
	WEIGHT						
	REPS						
	WEIGHT						
	REPS						
	WEIGHT						
	REPS						
	WEIGHT						

EXERCISE	SET	1	2	3	4	5	6
	REPS						
	WEIGHT						
	REPS						
	WEIGHT						
	REPS						
	WEIGHT						
	REPS						
	WEIGHT						
	REPS						
	WEIGHT						
	REPS						
	WEIGHT						

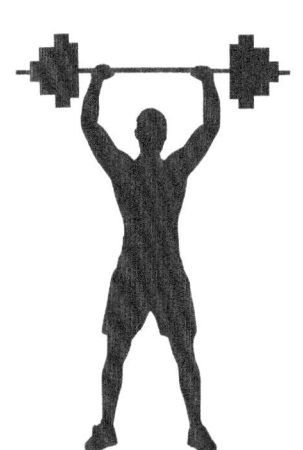

MEASUREMENTS	
NECK	
R BICEP	
L BICEP	
CHEST	
WAIST	
HIPS	
R THIGH	
L THIGH	
CALF	

NOTES

....
....
....
....
....
....
....
....
....
....

Workout Log Book

Date ....

WEIGHT   MON / TUE / WED / THU / FRI / SAT / SUN

MUSCLE GROUP   HOW I FEEL   1 / 2 / 3 / 4 / 5 / 6

START TIME   FINISH TIME

WATER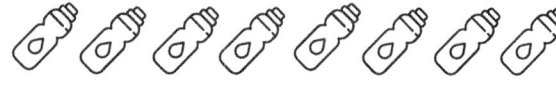

STRENGTH TRAINING

☐ UPPER BODY   ☐ LOWER BODY   ☐ ABS

CARDIO

EXERCISE	TIME	DISTANCE	CALS BURNED

EXERCISE	SET	1	2	3	4	5	6
	REPS						
	WEIGHT						
	REPS						
	WEIGHT						
	REPS						
	WEIGHT						
	REPS						
	WEIGHT						
	REPS						
	WEIGHT						
	REPS						
	WEIGHT						

EXERCISE	SET	1	2	3	4	5	6
	REPS						
	WEIGHT						
	REPS						
	WEIGHT						
	REPS						
	WEIGHT						
	REPS						
	WEIGHT						
	REPS						
	WEIGHT						
	REPS						
	WEIGHT						

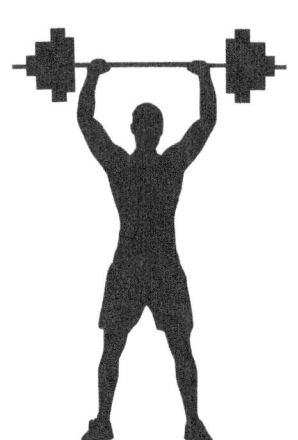

MEASUREMENTS	
NECK	
R BICEP	
L BICEP	
CHEST	
WAIST	
HIPS	
R THIGH	
L THIGH	
CALF	

NOTES

....
....
....
....
....
....
....
....
....
....
....

Workout Log Book

Date ....

WEIGHT MON / TUE / WED / THU / FRI / SAT / SUN

MUSCLE GROUP HOW I FEEL 1 / 2 / 3 / 4 / 5 / 6

START TIME FINISH TIME

WATER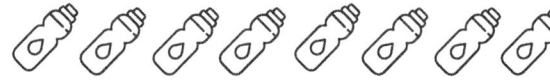

STRENGTH TRAINING

☐ UPPER BODY   ☐ LOWER BODY   ☐ ABS

CARDIO

EXERCISE	TIME	DISTANCE	CALS BURNED

EXERCISE	SET	1	2	3	4	5	6
	REPS						
	WEIGHT						
	REPS						
	WEIGHT						
	REPS						
	WEIGHT						
	REPS						
	WEIGHT						
	REPS						
	WEIGHT						
	REPS						
	WEIGHT						

EXERCISE	SET	1	2	3	4	5	6
	REPS						
	WEIGHT						
	REPS						
	WEIGHT						
	REPS						
	WEIGHT						
	REPS						
	WEIGHT						
	REPS						
	WEIGHT						
	REPS						
	WEIGHT						

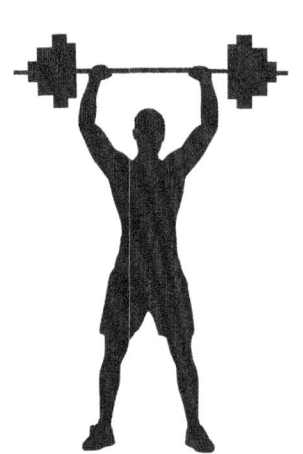

MEASUREMENTS	
NECK	
R BICEP	
L BICEP	
CHEST	
WAIST	
HIPS	
R THIGH	
L THIGH	
CALF	

NOTES

....
....
....
....
....
....
....
....
....
....
....

Workout Log Book

Date ....

WEIGHT

MON / TUE / WED / THU / FRI / SAT / SUN

MUSCLE GROUP

HOW I FEEL   1 / 2 / 3 / 4 / 5 / 6

START TIME   **FINISH TIME**

WATER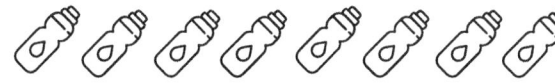

STRENGTH TRAINING

☐ UPPER BODY   ☐ LOWER BODY   ☐ ABS

CARDIO

EXERCISE	TIME	DISTANCE	CALS BURNED

EXERCISE	SET	1	2	3	4	5	6
	REPS						
	WEIGHT						
	REPS						
	WEIGHT						
	REPS						
	WEIGHT						
	REPS						
	WEIGHT						
	REPS						
	WEIGHT						
	REPS						
	WEIGHT						

EXERCISE	SET	1	2	3	4	5	6
	REPS						
	WEIGHT						
	REPS						
	WEIGHT						
	REPS						
	WEIGHT						
	REPS						
	WEIGHT						
	REPS						
	WEIGHT						
	REPS						
	WEIGHT						

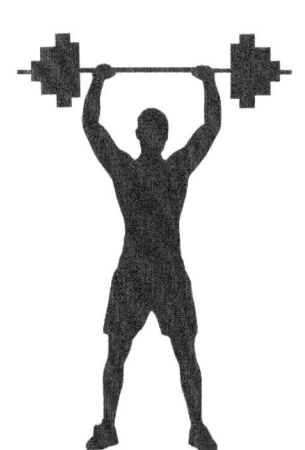

MEASUREMENTS	
NECK	
R BICEP	
L BICEP	
CHEST	
WAIST	
HIPS	
R THIGH	
L THIGH	
CALF	

NOTES

....
....
....
....
....
....
....
....
....
....
....

Workout Log Book

Date ....

WEIGHT MON / TUE / WED / THU / FRI / SAT / SUN

MUSCLE GROUP HOW I FEEL 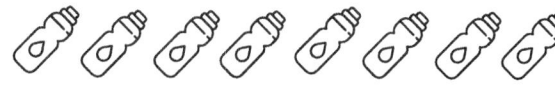 1 / 2 / 3 / 4 / 5 / 6

START TIME FINISH TIME

WATER 🍶🍶🍶🍶🍶🍶🍶

STRENGTH TRAINING

☐ UPPER BODY ☐ LOWER BODY ☐ ABS

CARDIO

EXERCISE	TIME	DISTANCE	CALS BURNED

EXERCISE	SET	1	2	3	4	5	6
	REPS						
	WEIGHT						
	REPS						
	WEIGHT						
	REPS						
	WEIGHT						
	REPS						
	WEIGHT						
	REPS						
	WEIGHT						
	REPS						
	WEIGHT						

EXERCISE	SET	1	2	3	4	5	6
	REPS						
	WEIGHT						
	REPS						
	WEIGHT						
	REPS						
	WEIGHT						
	REPS						
	WEIGHT						
	REPS						
	WEIGHT						
	REPS						
	WEIGHT						

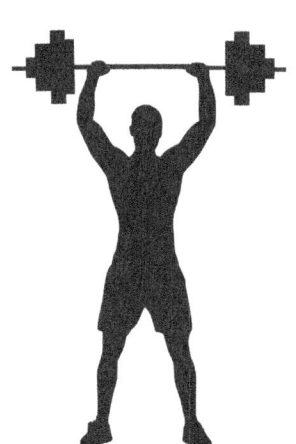

MEASUREMENTS	
NECK	
R BICEP	
L BICEP	
CHEST	
WAIST	
HIPS	
R THIGH	
L THIGH	
CALF	

NOTES

....
....
....
....
....
....
....
....
....
....
....
....

Workout Log Book

Date ....

WEIGHT　　　　　　MON / TUE / WED / THU / FRI / SAT / SUN

MUSCLE GROUP　　HOW I FEEL　1 / 2 / 3 / 4 / 5 / 6

START TIME　　　　FINISH TIME

WATER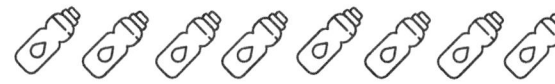

STRENGTH TRAINING

☐ UPPER BODY　　☐ LOWER BODY　　☐ ABS

CARDIO

EXERCISE	TIME	DISTANCE	CALS BURNED

EXERCISE	SET	1	2	3	4	5	6
	REPS						
	WEIGHT						
	REPS						
	WEIGHT						
	REPS						
	WEIGHT						
	REPS						
	WEIGHT						
	REPS						
	WEIGHT						
	REPS						
	WEIGHT						

EXERCISE	SET	1	2	3	4	5	6
	REPS						
	WEIGHT						
	REPS						
	WEIGHT						
	REPS						
	WEIGHT						
	REPS						
	WEIGHT						
	REPS						
	WEIGHT						
	REPS						
	WEIGHT						

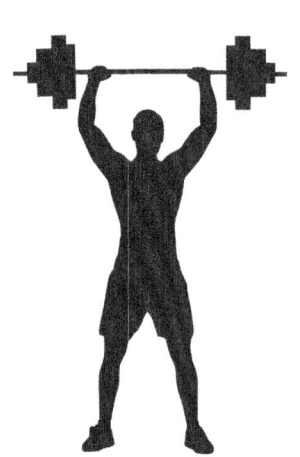

MEASUREMENTS	
NECK	
R BICEP	
L BICEP	
CHEST	
WAIST	
HIPS	
R THIGH	
L THIGH	
CALF	

NOTES

....
....
....
....
....
....
....
....
....
....

Workout Log Book

Date ....

WEIGHT   MON / TUE / WED / THU / FRI / SAT / SUN

MUSCLE GROUP   HOW I FEEL   1 / 2 / 3 / 4 / 5 / 6

START TIME   FINISH TIME

WATER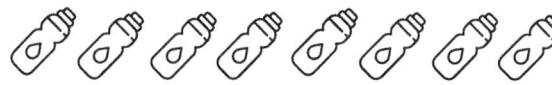

STRENGTH TRAINING

☐ UPPER BODY   ☐ LOWER BODY   ☐ ABS

CARDIO

EXERCISE	TIME	DISTANCE	CALS BURNED

EXERCISE	SET	1	2	3	4	5	6
	REPS						
	WEIGHT						
	REPS						
	WEIGHT						
	REPS						
	WEIGHT						
	REPS						
	WEIGHT						
	REPS						
	WEIGHT						
	REPS						
	WEIGHT						

EXERCISE	SET	1	2	3	4	5	6
	REPS						
	WEIGHT						
	REPS						
	WEIGHT						
	REPS						
	WEIGHT						
	REPS						
	WEIGHT						
	REPS						
	WEIGHT						
	REPS						
	WEIGHT						

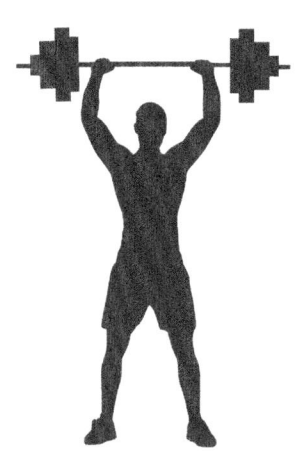

MEASUREMENTS	
NECK	
R BICEP	
L BICEP	
CHEST	
WAIST	
HIPS	
R THIGH	
L THIGH	
CALF	

NOTES

....
....
....
....
....
....
....
....
....
....

Workout Log Book

Date ....

WEIGHT MON / TUE / WED / THU / FRI / SAT / SUN

MUSCLE GROUP HOW I FEEL 1 / 2 / 3 / 4 / 5 / 6

START TIME FINISH TIME

WATER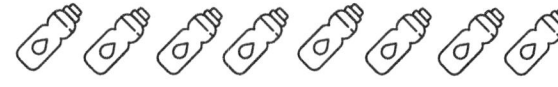

STRENGTH TRAINING

☐ UPPER BODY ☐ LOWER BODY ☐ ABS

CARDIO

EXERCISE	TIME	DISTANCE	CALS BURNED

EXERCISE	SET	1	2	3	4	5	6
	REPS						
	WEIGHT						
	REPS						
	WEIGHT						
	REPS						
	WEIGHT						
	REPS						
	WEIGHT						
	REPS						
	WEIGHT						
	REPS						
	WEIGHT						

EXERCISE	SET	1	2	3	4	5	6
	REPS						
	WEIGHT						
	REPS						
	WEIGHT						
	REPS						
	WEIGHT						
	REPS						
	WEIGHT						
	REPS						
	WEIGHT						
	REPS						
	WEIGHT						

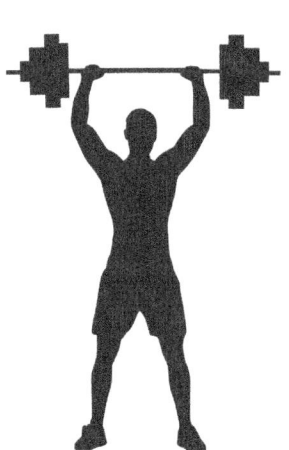

MEASUREMENTS	
NECK	
R BICEP	
L BICEP	
CHEST	
WAIST	
HIPS	
R THIGH	
L THIGH	
CALF	

NOTES

....
....
....
....
....
....
....
....
....
....
....
....

Workout Log Book

Date ....

WEIGHT　　　　　　　MON / TUE / WED / THU / FRI / SAT / SUN

MUSCLE GROUP　　　HOW I FEEL　1 / 2 / 3 / 4 / 5 / 6

START TIME　　　　　FINISH TIME

WATER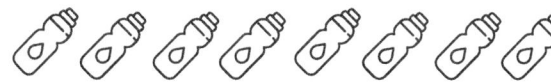

STRENGTH TRAINING

☐ UPPER BODY　　☐ LOWER BODY　　☐ ABS

CARDIO

EXERCISE	TIME	DISTANCE	CALS BURNED

EXERCISE	SET	1	2	3	4	5	6
	REPS						
	WEIGHT						
	REPS						
	WEIGHT						
	REPS						
	WEIGHT						
	REPS						
	WEIGHT						
	REPS						
	WEIGHT						
	REPS						
	WEIGHT						

EXERCISE	SET	1	2	3	4	5	6
	REPS						
	WEIGHT						
	REPS						
	WEIGHT						
	REPS						
	WEIGHT						
	REPS						
	WEIGHT						
	REPS						
	WEIGHT						
	REPS						
	WEIGHT						

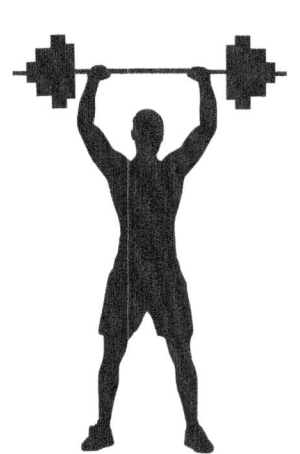

MEASUREMENTS	
NECK	
R BICEP	
L BICEP	
CHEST	
WAIST	
HIPS	
R THIGH	
L THIGH	
CALF	

NOTES

....
....
....
....
....
....
....
....
....
....

Workout Log Book

Date ....

WEIGHT MON / TUE / WED / THU / FRI / SAT / SUN

MUSCLE GROUP HOW I FEEL 1 / 2 / 3 / 4 / 5 / 6

START TIME FINISH TIME

WATER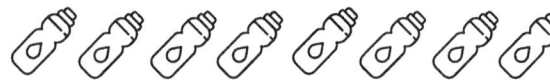

STRENGTH TRAINING

☐ UPPER BODY ☐ LOWER BODY ☐ ABS

CARDIO

EXERCISE	TIME	DISTANCE	CALS BURNED

EXERCISE	SET	1	2	3	4	5	6
	REPS						
	WEIGHT						
	REPS						
	WEIGHT						
	REPS						
	WEIGHT						
	REPS						
	WEIGHT						
	REPS						
	WEIGHT						
	REPS						
	WEIGHT						

EXERCISE	SET	1	2	3	4	5	6
	REPS						
	WEIGHT						
	REPS						
	WEIGHT						
	REPS						
	WEIGHT						
	REPS						
	WEIGHT						
	REPS						
	WEIGHT						
	REPS						
	WEIGHT						

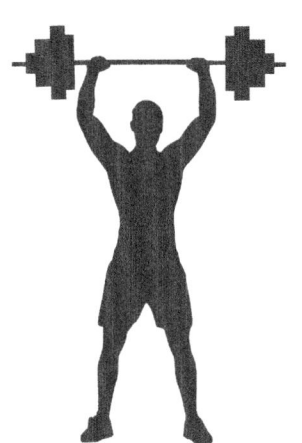

MEASUREMENTS	
NECK	
R BICEP	
L BICEP	
CHEST	
WAIST	
HIPS	
R THIGH	
L THIGH	
CALF	

NOTES

....
....
....
....
....
....
....
....
....
....

Workout Log Book

Date ....

WEIGHT MON / TUE / WED / THU / FRI / SAT / SUN

MUSCLE GROUP HOW I FEEL 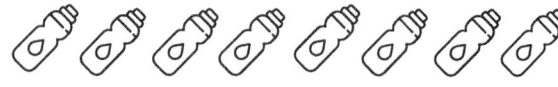 1 / 2 / 3 / 4 / 5 / 6

START TIME FINISH TIME

WATER 🍼🍼🍼🍼🍼🍼🍼🍼

STRENGTH TRAINING

☐ UPPER BODY ☐ LOWER BODY ☐ ABS

CARDIO

EXERCISE	TIME	DISTANCE	CALS BURNED

EXERCISE	SET	1	2	3	4	5	6
	REPS						
	WEIGHT						
	REPS						
	WEIGHT						
	REPS						
	WEIGHT						
	REPS						
	WEIGHT						
	REPS						
	WEIGHT						
	REPS						
	WEIGHT						

EXERCISE	SET	1	2	3	4	5	6
	REPS						
	WEIGHT						
	REPS						
	WEIGHT						
	REPS						
	WEIGHT						
	REPS						
	WEIGHT						
	REPS						
	WEIGHT						
	REPS						
	WEIGHT						

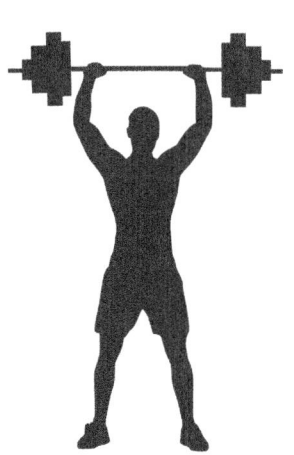

MEASUREMENTS	
NECK	
R BICEP	
L BICEP	
CHEST	
WAIST	
HIPS	
R THIGH	
L THIGH	
CALF	

NOTES

....
....
....
....
....
....
....
....
....
....
....

Workout Log Book

Date ....

WEIGHT

MUSCLE GROUP

START TIME

MON / TUE / WED / THU / FRI / SAT / SUN

HOW I FEEL   1 / 2 / 3 / 4 / 5 / 6

FINISH TIME

WATER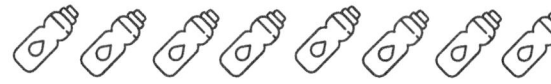

STRENGTH TRAINING

☐ UPPER BODY   ☐ LOWER BODY   ☐ ABS

CARDIO

EXERCISE	TIME	DISTANCE	CALS BURNED

EXERCISE	SET	1	2	3	4	5	6
	REPS						
	WEIGHT						
	REPS						
	WEIGHT						
	REPS						
	WEIGHT						
	REPS						
	WEIGHT						
	REPS						
	WEIGHT						
	REPS						
	WEIGHT						

EXERCISE	SET	1	2	3	4	5	6
	REPS						
	WEIGHT						
	REPS						
	WEIGHT						
	REPS						
	WEIGHT						
	REPS						
	WEIGHT						
	REPS						
	WEIGHT						
	REPS						
	WEIGHT						

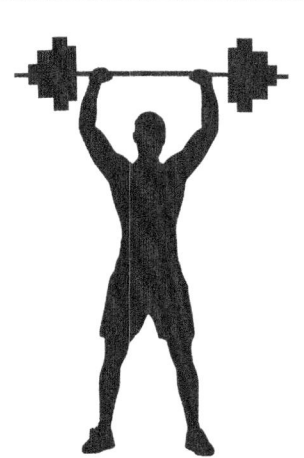

MEASUREMENTS	
NECK	
R BICEP	
L BICEP	
CHEST	
WAIST	
HIPS	
R THIGH	
L THIGH	
CALF	

NOTES

Workout Log Book

Date ....

WEIGHT MON / TUE / WED / THU / FRI / SAT / SUN

MUSCLE GROUP HOW I FEEL 1 / 2 / 3 / 4 / 5 / 6

START TIME FINISH TIME

WATER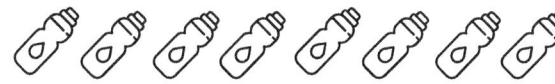

STRENGTH TRAINING

☐ UPPER BODY ☐ LOWER BODY ☐ ABS

CARDIO

EXERCISE	TIME	DISTANCE	CALS BURNED

EXERCISE	SET	1	2	3	4	5	6
	REPS						
	WEIGHT						
	REPS						
	WEIGHT						
	REPS						
	WEIGHT						
	REPS						
	WEIGHT						
	REPS						
	WEIGHT						
	REPS						
	WEIGHT						

EXERCISE	SET	1	2	3	4	5	6
	REPS						
	WEIGHT						
	REPS						
	WEIGHT						
	REPS						
	WEIGHT						
	REPS						
	WEIGHT						
	REPS						
	WEIGHT						
	REPS						
	WEIGHT						

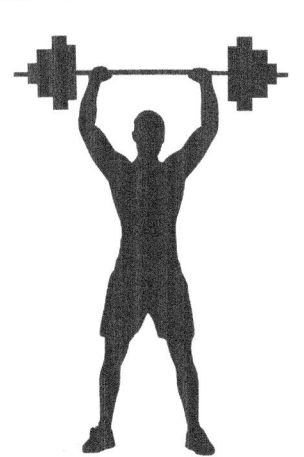

MEASUREMENTS	
NECK	
R BICEP	
L BICEP	
CHEST	
WAIST	
HIPS	
R THIGH	
L THIGH	
CALF	

NOTES

....
....
....
....
....
....
....
....
....
....
....

Workout Log Book

Date ....

WEIGHT MON / TUE / WED / THU / FRI / SAT / SUN

MUSCLE GROUP HOW I FEEL 1 / 2 / 3 / 4 / 5 / 6

START TIME FINISH TIME

WATER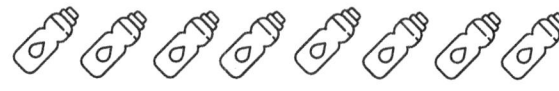

STRENGTH TRAINING

☐ UPPER BODY ☐ LOWER BODY ☐ ABS

CARDIO

EXERCISE	TIME	DISTANCE	CALS BURNED

EXERCISE	SET	1	2	3	4	5	6
	REPS						
	WEIGHT						
	REPS						
	WEIGHT						
	REPS						
	WEIGHT						
	REPS						
	WEIGHT						
	REPS						
	WEIGHT						
	REPS						
	WEIGHT						

EXERCISE	SET	1	2	3	4	5	6
	REPS						
	WEIGHT						
	REPS						
	WEIGHT						
	REPS						
	WEIGHT						
	REPS						
	WEIGHT						
	REPS						
	WEIGHT						
	REPS						
	WEIGHT						

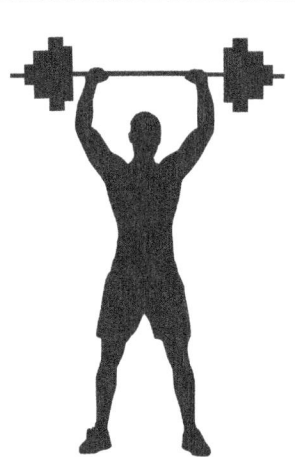

MEASUREMENTS	
NECK	
R BICEP	
L BICEP	
CHEST	
WAIST	
HIPS	
R THIGH	
L THIGH	
CALF	

NOTES

....
....
....
....
....
....
....
....
....
....
....

Workout Log Book

Date ....

WEIGHT MON / TUE / WED / THU / FRI / SAT / SUN

MUSCLE GROUP HOW I FEEL 1 / 2 / 3 / 4 / 5 / 6

START TIME FINISH TIME

WATER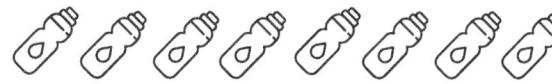

STRENGTH TRAINING

☐ UPPER BODY   ☐ LOWER BODY   ☐ ABS

CARDIO

EXERCISE	TIME	DISTANCE	CALS BURNED

EXERCISE	SET	1	2	3	4	5	6
	REPS						
	WEIGHT						
	REPS						
	WEIGHT						
	REPS						
	WEIGHT						
	REPS						
	WEIGHT						
	REPS						
	WEIGHT						
	REPS						
	WEIGHT						

EXERCISE	SET	1	2	3	4	5	6
	REPS						
	WEIGHT						
	REPS						
	WEIGHT						
	REPS						
	WEIGHT						
	REPS						
	WEIGHT						
	REPS						
	WEIGHT						
	REPS						
	WEIGHT						

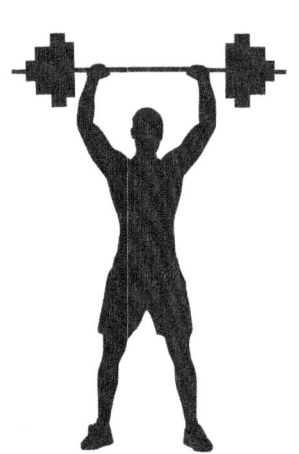

MEASUREMENTS	
NECK	
R BICEP	
L BICEP	
CHEST	
WAIST	
HIPS	
R THIGH	
L THIGH	
CALF	

NOTES

....
....
....
....
....
....
....
....
....
....

Workout Log Book

Date ....

WEIGHT　　　　　　　MON / TUE / WED / THU / FRI / SAT / SUN

MUSCLE GROUP　　　　　HOW I FEEL　　1 / 2 / 3 / 4 / 5 / 6

START TIME　　　　　　FINISH TIME

WATER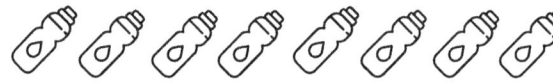

STRENGTH TRAINING

☐ UPPER BODY　　☐ LOWER BODY　　☐ ABS

CARDIO

EXERCISE	TIME	DISTANCE	CALS BURNED

EXERCISE	SET	1	2	3	4	5	6
	REPS						
	WEIGHT						
	REPS						
	WEIGHT						
	REPS						
	WEIGHT						
	REPS						
	WEIGHT						
	REPS						
	WEIGHT						
	REPS						
	WEIGHT						

EXERCISE	SET	1	2	3	4	5	6
	REPS						
	WEIGHT						
	REPS						
	WEIGHT						
	REPS						
	WEIGHT						
	REPS						
	WEIGHT						
	REPS						
	WEIGHT						
	REPS						
	WEIGHT						

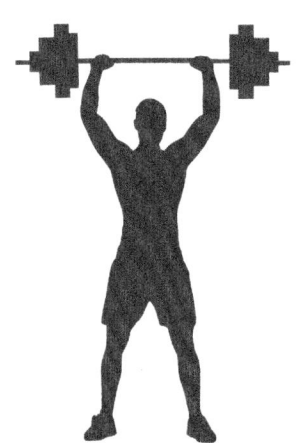

MEASUREMENTS	
NECK	
R BICEP	
L BICEP	
CHEST	
WAIST	
HIPS	
R THIGH	
L THIGH	
CALF	

NOTES

....
....
....
....
....
....
....
....
....
....
....

Workout Log Book

Date ....

WEIGHT MON / TUE / WED / THU / FRI / SAT / SUN

MUSCLE GROUP HOW I FEEL 1 / 2 / 3 / 4 / 5 / 6

START TIME FINISH TIME

WATER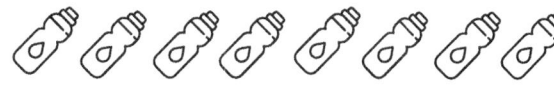

STRENGTH TRAINING

☐ UPPER BODY ☐ LOWER BODY ☐ ABS

CARDIO

EXERCISE	TIME	DISTANCE	CALS BURNED

EXERCISE	SET	1	2	3	4	5	6
	REPS						
	WEIGHT						
	REPS						
	WEIGHT						
	REPS						
	WEIGHT						
	REPS						
	WEIGHT						
	REPS						
	WEIGHT						
	REPS						
	WEIGHT						

EXERCISE	SET	1	2	3	4	5	6
	REPS						
	WEIGHT						
	REPS						
	WEIGHT						
	REPS						
	WEIGHT						
	REPS						
	WEIGHT						
	REPS						
	WEIGHT						
	REPS						
	WEIGHT						

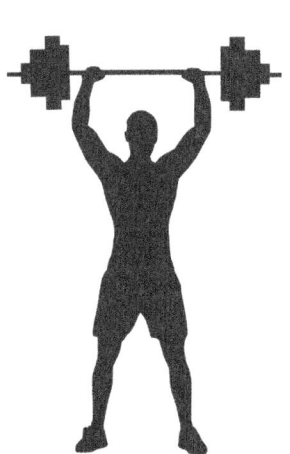

MEASUREMENTS	
NECK	
R BICEP	
L BICEP	
CHEST	
WAIST	
HIPS	
R THIGH	
L THIGH	
CALF	

NOTES

....
....
....
....
....
....
....
....
....
....

Workout Log Book

Date ....

WEIGHT MON / TUE / WED / THU / FRI / SAT / SUN

MUSCLE GROUP HOW I FEEL 1 / 2 / 3 / 4 / 5 / 6

START TIME FINISH TIME

WATER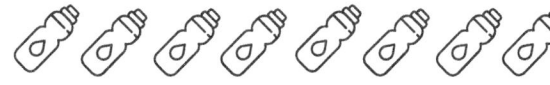

STRENGTH TRAINING

☐ UPPER BODY ☐ LOWER BODY ☐ ABS

CARDIO

EXERCISE	TIME	DISTANCE	CALS BURNED

EXERCISE	SET	1	2	3	4	5	6
	REPS						
	WEIGHT						
	REPS						
	WEIGHT						
	REPS						
	WEIGHT						
	REPS						
	WEIGHT						
	REPS						
	WEIGHT						
	REPS						
	WEIGHT						

EXERCISE	SET	1	2	3	4	5	6
	REPS						
	WEIGHT						
	REPS						
	WEIGHT						
	REPS						
	WEIGHT						
	REPS						
	WEIGHT						
	REPS						
	WEIGHT						
	REPS						
	WEIGHT						

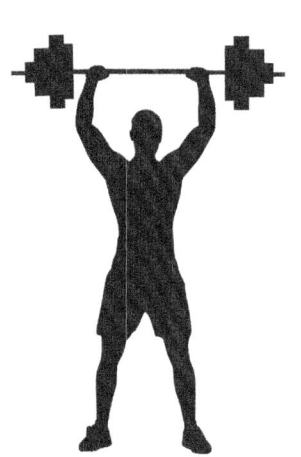

MEASUREMENTS	
NECK	
R BICEP	
L BICEP	
CHEST	
WAIST	
HIPS	
R THIGH	
L THIGH	
CALF	

NOTES

....
....
....
....
....
....
....
....
....
....

Workout Log Book

Date ....

WEIGHT MON / TUE / WED / THU / FRI / SAT / SUN

MUSCLE GROUP HOW I FEEL 1 / 2 / 3 / 4 / 5 / 6

START TIME FINISH TIME

WATER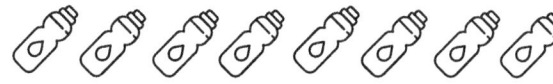

STRENGTH TRAINING

☐ UPPER BODY ☐ LOWER BODY ☐ ABS

CARDIO

EXERCISE	TIME	DISTANCE	CALS BURNED

EXERCISE	SET	1	2	3	4	5	6
	REPS						
	WEIGHT						
	REPS						
	WEIGHT						
	REPS						
	WEIGHT						
	REPS						
	WEIGHT						
	REPS						
	WEIGHT						
	REPS						
	WEIGHT						

EXERCISE	SET	1	2	3	4	5	6
	REPS						
	WEIGHT						
	REPS						
	WEIGHT						
	REPS						
	WEIGHT						
	REPS						
	WEIGHT						
	REPS						
	WEIGHT						
	REPS						
	WEIGHT						

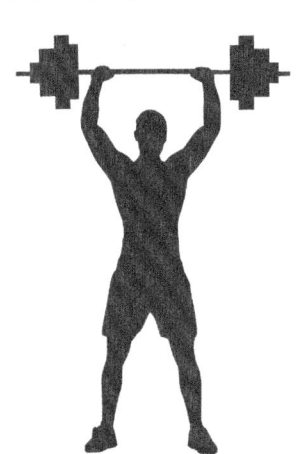

MEASUREMENTS	
NECK	
R BICEP	
L BICEP	
CHEST	
WAIST	
HIPS	
R THIGH	
L THIGH	
CALF	

NOTES

....
....
....
....
....
....
....
....
....
....
....

Workout Log Book

Date ....

WEIGHT MON / TUE / WED / THU / FRI / SAT / SUN

MUSCLE GROUP HOW I FEEL 1 / 2 / 3 / 4 / 5 / 6

START TIME FINISH TIME

WATER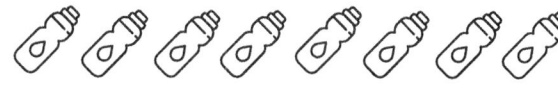

STRENGTH TRAINING

☐ UPPER BODY ☐ LOWER BODY ☐ ABS

CARDIO

EXERCISE	TIME	DISTANCE	CALS BURNED

EXERCISE	SET	1	2	3	4	5	6
	REPS						
	WEIGHT						
	REPS						
	WEIGHT						
	REPS						
	WEIGHT						
	REPS						
	WEIGHT						
	REPS						
	WEIGHT						
	REPS						
	WEIGHT						

EXERCISE	SET	1	2	3	4	5	6
	REPS						
	WEIGHT						
	REPS						
	WEIGHT						
	REPS						
	WEIGHT						
	REPS						
	WEIGHT						
	REPS						
	WEIGHT						
	REPS						
	WEIGHT						

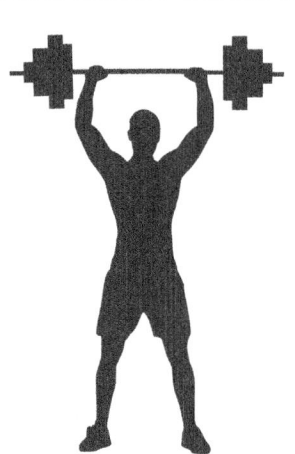

MEASUREMENTS	
NECK	
R BICEP	
L BICEP	
CHEST	
WAIST	
HIPS	
R THIGH	
L THIGH	
CALF	

NOTES

....
....
....
....
....
....
....
....
....
....

Workout Log Book

Date ....

WEIGHT

MUSCLE GROUP

START TIME

MON / TUE / WED / THU / FRI / SAT / SUN

HOW I FEEL   1 / 2 / 3 / 4 / 5 / 6

FINISH TIME

WATER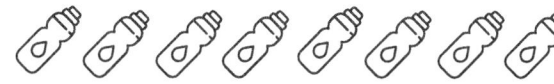

STRENGTH TRAINING

☐ UPPER BODY   ☐ LOWER BODY   ☐ ABS

CARDIO

EXERCISE	TIME	DISTANCE	CALS BURNED

EXERCISE	SET	1	2	3	4	5	6
	REPS						
	WEIGHT						
	REPS						
	WEIGHT						
	REPS						
	WEIGHT						
	REPS						
	WEIGHT						
	REPS						
	WEIGHT						
	REPS						
	WEIGHT						

EXERCISE	SET	1	2	3	4	5	6
	REPS						
	WEIGHT						
	REPS						
	WEIGHT						
	REPS						
	WEIGHT						
	REPS						
	WEIGHT						
	REPS						
	WEIGHT						
	REPS						
	WEIGHT						

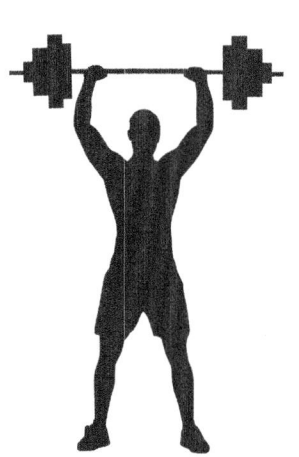

MEASUREMENTS	
NECK	
R BICEP	
L BICEP	
CHEST	
WAIST	
HIPS	
R THIGH	
L THIGH	
CALF	

NOTES

....
....
....
....
....
....
....
....
....
....

Workout Log Book

Date ....

WEIGHT   MON / TUE / WED / THU / FRI / SAT / SUN

MUSCLE GROUP   HOW I FEEL   1 / 2 / 3 / 4 / 5 / 6

START TIME   FINISH TIME

WATER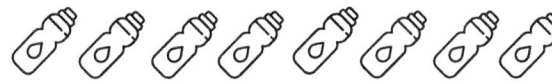

STRENGTH TRAINING

☐ UPPER BODY   ☐ LOWER BODY   ☐ ABS

CARDIO

EXERCISE	TIME	DISTANCE	CALS BURNED

EXERCISE	SET	1	2	3	4	5	6
	REPS						
	WEIGHT						
	REPS						
	WEIGHT						
	REPS						
	WEIGHT						
	REPS						
	WEIGHT						
	REPS						
	WEIGHT						
	REPS						
	WEIGHT						

EXERCISE	SET	1	2	3	4	5	6
	REPS						
	WEIGHT						
	REPS						
	WEIGHT						
	REPS						
	WEIGHT						
	REPS						
	WEIGHT						
	REPS						
	WEIGHT						
	REPS						
	WEIGHT						

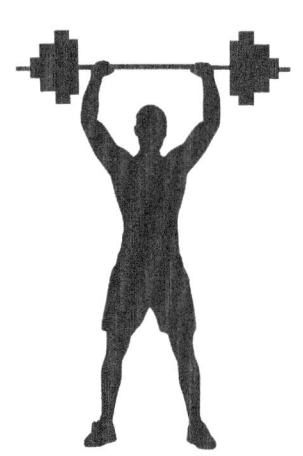

MEASUREMENTS	
NECK	
R BICEP	
L BICEP	
CHEST	
WAIST	
HIPS	
R THIGH	
L THIGH	
CALF	

NOTES

....
....
....
....
....
....
....
....
....
....

Workout Log Book

Date ....

WEIGHT MON / TUE / WED / THU / FRI / SAT / SUN

MUSCLE GROUP HOW I FEEL 1 / 2 / 3 / 4 / 5 / 6

START TIME FINISH TIME

WATER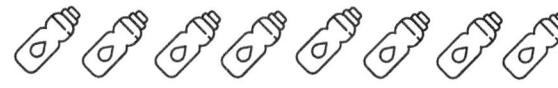

STRENGTH TRAINING

☐ UPPER BODY ☐ LOWER BODY ☐ ABS

CARDIO

EXERCISE	TIME	DISTANCE	CALS BURNED

EXERCISE	SET	1	2	3	4	5	6
	REPS						
	WEIGHT						
	REPS						
	WEIGHT						
	REPS						
	WEIGHT						
	REPS						
	WEIGHT						
	REPS						
	WEIGHT						
	REPS						
	WEIGHT						

EXERCISE	SET	1	2	3	4	5	6
	REPS						
	WEIGHT						
	REPS						
	WEIGHT						
	REPS						
	WEIGHT						
	REPS						
	WEIGHT						
	REPS						
	WEIGHT						
	REPS						
	WEIGHT						

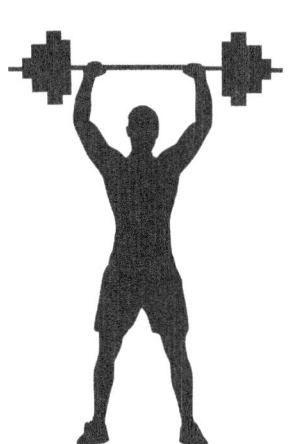

MEASUREMENTS	
NECK	
R BICEP	
L BICEP	
CHEST	
WAIST	
HIPS	
R THIGH	
L THIGH	
CALF	

NOTES

....
....
....
....
....
....
....
....
....
....

Workout Log Book

Date ....

WEIGHT   MON / TUE / WED / THU / FRI / SAT / SUN

MUSCLE GROUP   HOW I FEEL   1 / 2 / 3 / 4 / 5 / 6

START TIME   FINISH TIME

WATER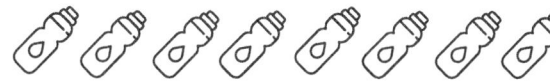

STRENGTH TRAINING

☐ UPPER BODY   ☐ LOWER BODY   ☐ ABS

CARDIO

EXERCISE	TIME	DISTANCE	CALS BURNED

EXERCISE	SET	1	2	3	4	5	6
	REPS						
	WEIGHT						
	REPS						
	WEIGHT						
	REPS						
	WEIGHT						
	REPS						
	WEIGHT						
	REPS						
	WEIGHT						

EXERCISE	SET	1	2	3	4	5	6
	REPS						
	WEIGHT						
	REPS						
	WEIGHT						
	REPS						
	WEIGHT						
	REPS						
	WEIGHT						
	REPS						
	WEIGHT						
	REPS						
	WEIGHT						

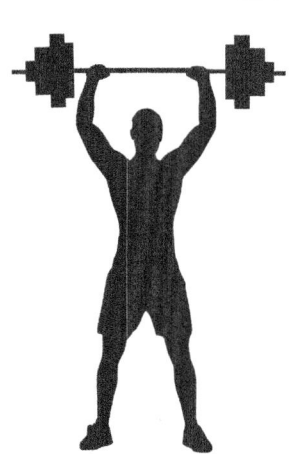

MEASUREMENTS	
NECK	
R BICEP	
L BICEP	
CHEST	
WAIST	
HIPS	
R THIGH	
L THIGH	
CALF	

NOTES

....
....
....
....
....
....
....
....
....
....
....

Workout Log Book

Date ....

WEIGHT MON / TUE / WED / THU / FRI / SAT / SUN

MUSCLE GROUP HOW I FEEL 1 / 2 / 3 / 4 / 5 / 6

START TIME FINISH TIME

WATER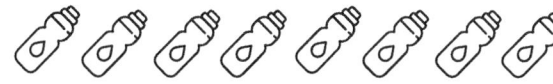

STRENGTH TRAINING

☐ UPPER BODY ☐ LOWER BODY ☐ ABS

CARDIO

EXERCISE	TIME	DISTANCE	CALS BURNED

EXERCISE	SET	1	2	3	4	5	6
	REPS						
	WEIGHT						
	REPS						
	WEIGHT						
	REPS						
	WEIGHT						
	REPS						
	WEIGHT						
	REPS						
	WEIGHT						
	REPS						
	WEIGHT						

EXERCISE	SET	1	2	3	4	5	6
	REPS						
	WEIGHT						
	REPS						
	WEIGHT						
	REPS						
	WEIGHT						
	REPS						
	WEIGHT						
	REPS						
	WEIGHT						
	REPS						
	WEIGHT						

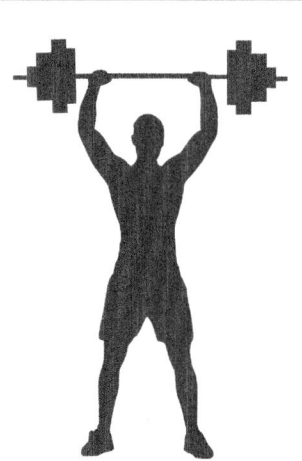

MEASUREMENTS	
NECK	
R BICEP	
L BICEP	
CHEST	
WAIST	
HIPS	
R THIGH	
L THIGH	
CALF	

NOTES

....
....
....
....
....
....
....
....
....
....

Workout Log Book

Date ....

WEIGHT MON / TUE / WED / THU / FRI / SAT / SUN

MUSCLE GROUP HOW I FEEL 1 / 2 / 3 / 4 / 5 / 6

START TIME FINISH TIME

WATER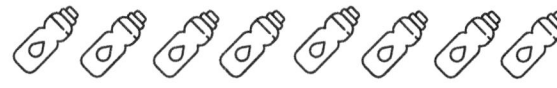

STRENGTH TRAINING

☐ UPPER BODY   ☐ LOWER BODY   ☐ ABS

CARDIO

EXERCISE	TIME	DISTANCE	CALS BURNED

EXERCISE	SET	1	2	3	4	5	6
	REPS						
	WEIGHT						
	REPS						
	WEIGHT						
	REPS						
	WEIGHT						
	REPS						
	WEIGHT						
	REPS						
	WEIGHT						
	REPS						
	WEIGHT						

EXERCISE	SET	1	2	3	4	5	6
	REPS						
	WEIGHT						
	REPS						
	WEIGHT						
	REPS						
	WEIGHT						
	REPS						
	WEIGHT						
	REPS						
	WEIGHT						
	REPS						
	WEIGHT						

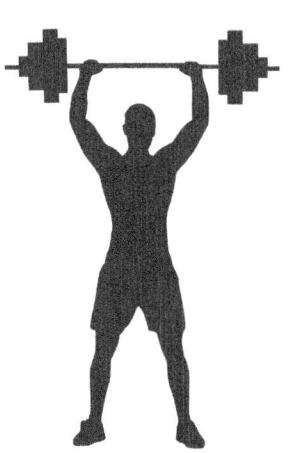

MEASUREMENTS	
NECK	
R BICEP	
L BICEP	
CHEST	
WAIST	
HIPS	
R THIGH	
L THIGH	
CALF	

NOTES

....
....
....
....
....
....
....
....
....
....
....

Workout Log Book

Date ....

WEIGHT MON / TUE / WED / THU / FRI / SAT / SUN

MUSCLE GROUP HOW I FEEL 1 / 2 / 3 / 4 / 5 / 6

START TIME FINISH TIME

WATER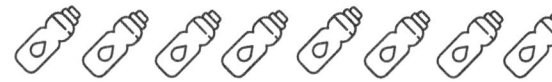

STRENGTH TRAINING

☐ UPPER BODY ☐ LOWER BODY ☐ ABS

CARDIO

EXERCISE	TIME	DISTANCE	CALS BURNED

EXERCISE	SET	1	2	3	4	5	6
	REPS						
	WEIGHT						
	REPS						
	WEIGHT						
	REPS						
	WEIGHT						
	REPS						
	WEIGHT						
	REPS						
	WEIGHT						
	REPS						
	WEIGHT						

EXERCISE	SET	1	2	3	4	5	6
	REPS						
	WEIGHT						
	REPS						
	WEIGHT						
	REPS						
	WEIGHT						
	REPS						
	WEIGHT						
	REPS						
	WEIGHT						
	REPS						
	WEIGHT						

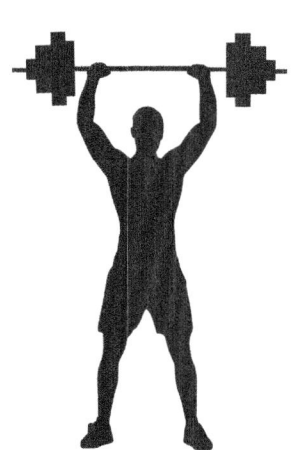

MEASUREMENTS	
NECK	
R BICEP	
L BICEP	
CHEST	
WAIST	
HIPS	
R THIGH	
L THIGH	
CALF	

NOTES

....
....
....
....
....
....
....
....
....
....
....

Workout Log Book

Date ....

WEIGHT MON / TUE / WED / THU / FRI / SAT / SUN

MUSCLE GROUP HOW I FEEL 1 / 2 / 3 / 4 / 5 / 6

START TIME FINISH TIME

WATER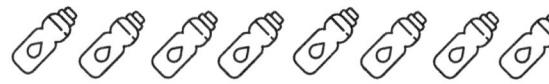

STRENGTH TRAINING

☐ UPPER BODY ☐ LOWER BODY ☐ ABS

CARDIO

EXERCISE	TIME	DISTANCE	CALS BURNED

EXERCISE	SET	1	2	3	4	5	6
	REPS						
	WEIGHT						
	REPS						
	WEIGHT						
	REPS						
	WEIGHT						
	REPS						
	WEIGHT						
	REPS						
	WEIGHT						
	REPS						
	WEIGHT						

EXERCISE	SET	1	2	3	4	5	6
	REPS						
	WEIGHT						
	REPS						
	WEIGHT						
	REPS						
	WEIGHT						
	REPS						
	WEIGHT						
	REPS						
	WEIGHT						
	REPS						
	WEIGHT						

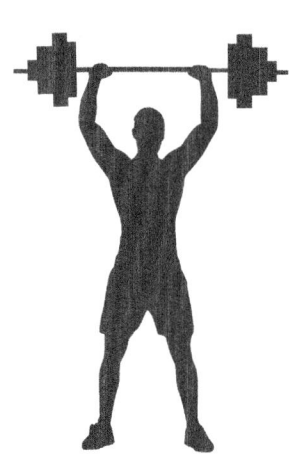

MEASUREMENTS	
NECK	
R BICEP	
L BICEP	
CHEST	
WAIST	
HIPS	
R THIGH	
L THIGH	
CALF	

NOTES

....
....
....
....
....
....
....
....
....
....
....

Workout Log Book

Date ....

WEIGHT　　　　　MON / TUE / WED / THU / FRI / SAT / SUN

MUSCLE GROUP　　　　HOW I FEEL　　1 / 2 / 3 / 4 / 5 / 6

START TIME　　　　　FINISH TIME

WATER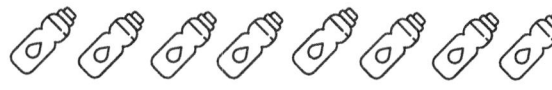

STRENGTH TRAINING

☐ UPPER BODY　　☐ LOWER BODY　　☐ ABS

CARDIO

EXERCISE	TIME	DISTANCE	CALS BURNED

EXERCISE	SET	1	2	3	4	5	6
	REPS						
	WEIGHT						
	REPS						
	WEIGHT						
	REPS						
	WEIGHT						
	REPS						
	WEIGHT						
	REPS						
	WEIGHT						
	REPS						
	WEIGHT						

EXERCISE	SET	1	2	3	4	5	6
	REPS						
	WEIGHT						
	REPS						
	WEIGHT						
	REPS						
	WEIGHT						
	REPS						
	WEIGHT						
	REPS						
	WEIGHT						
	REPS						
	WEIGHT						

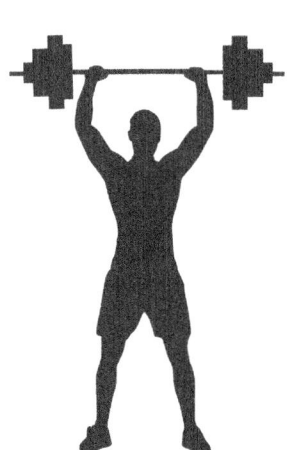

MEASUREMENTS	
NECK	
R BICEP	
L BICEP	
CHEST	
WAIST	
HIPS	
R THIGH	
L THIGH	
CALF	

NOTES

....
....
....
....
....
....
....
....
....
....

Workout Log Book

Date ....

WEIGHT   MON / TUE / WED / THU / FRI / SAT / SUN

MUSCLE GROUP   HOW I FEEL   1 / 2 / 3 / 4 / 5 / 6

START TIME   FINISH TIME

WATER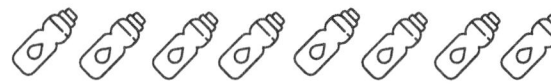

STRENGTH TRAINING

☐ UPPER BODY   ☐ LOWER BODY   ☐ ABS

CARDIO

EXERCISE	TIME	DISTANCE	CALS BURNED

EXERCISE	SET	1	2	3	4	5	6
	REPS						
	WEIGHT						
	REPS						
	WEIGHT						
	REPS						
	WEIGHT						
	REPS						
	WEIGHT						
	REPS						
	WEIGHT						
	REPS						
	WEIGHT						

EXERCISE	SET	1	2	3	4	5	6
	REPS						
	WEIGHT						
	REPS						
	WEIGHT						
	REPS						
	WEIGHT						
	REPS						
	WEIGHT						
	REPS						
	WEIGHT						
	REPS						
	WEIGHT						

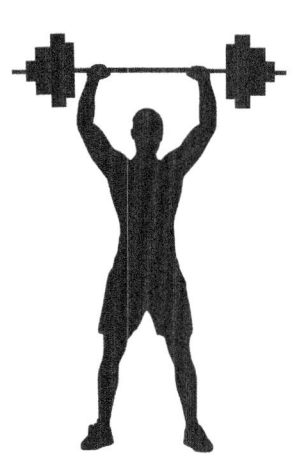

MEASUREMENTS	
NECK	
R BICEP	
L BICEP	
CHEST	
WAIST	
HIPS	
R THIGH	
L THIGH	
CALF	

NOTES

....
....
....
....
....
....
....
....
....
....

Workout Log Book

Date ....

WEIGHT

MUSCLE GROUP

START TIME   **FINISH TIME**

MON / TUE / WED / THU / FRI / SAT / SUN

HOW I FEEL 1 / 2 / 3 / 4 / 5 / 6

WATER

STRENGTH TRAINING

☐ UPPER BODY   ☐ LOWER BODY   ☐ ABS

CARDIO

EXERCISE	TIME	DISTANCE	CALS BURNED

EXERCISE	SET	1	2	3	4	5	6
	REPS						
	WEIGHT						
	REPS						
	WEIGHT						
	REPS						
	WEIGHT						
	REPS						
	WEIGHT						
	REPS						
	WEIGHT						
	REPS						
	WEIGHT						

EXERCISE	SET	1	2	3	4	5	6
	REPS						
	WEIGHT						
	REPS						
	WEIGHT						
	REPS						
	WEIGHT						
	REPS						
	WEIGHT						
	REPS						
	WEIGHT						
	REPS						
	WEIGHT						

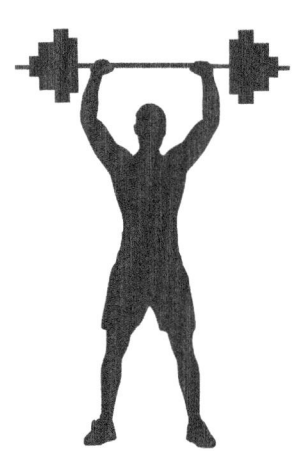

MEASUREMENTS	
NECK	
R BICEP	
L BICEP	
CHEST	
WAIST	
HIPS	
R THIGH	
L THIGH	
CALF	

NOTES

....
....
....
....
....
....
....
....
....
....
....
....

Workout Log Book

Date ....

WEIGHT　　　　　　MON / TUE / WED / THU / FRI / SAT / SUN

MUSCLE GROUP　　　HOW I FEEL　 1 / 2 / 3 / 4 / 5 / 6

START TIME　　　　　FINISH TIME

WATER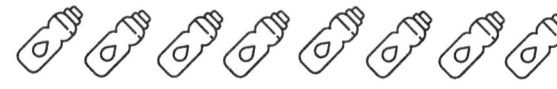

STRENGTH TRAINING

☐ UPPER BODY　　☐ LOWER BODY　　☐ ABS

CARDIO

EXERCISE	TIME	DISTANCE	CALS BURNED

EXERCISE	SET	1	2	3	4	5	6
	REPS						
	WEIGHT						
	REPS						
	WEIGHT						
	REPS						
	WEIGHT						
	REPS						
	WEIGHT						
	REPS						
	WEIGHT						
	REPS						
	WEIGHT						

EXERCISE	SET	1	2	3	4	5	6
	REPS						
	WEIGHT						
	REPS						
	WEIGHT						
	REPS						
	WEIGHT						
	REPS						
	WEIGHT						
	REPS						
	WEIGHT						
	REPS						
	WEIGHT						

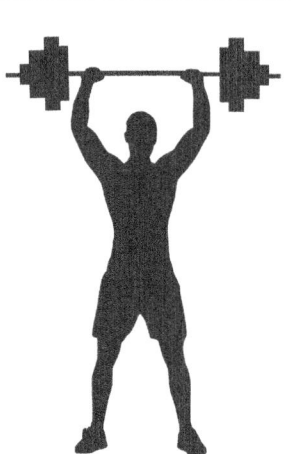

MEASUREMENTS	
NECK	
R BICEP	
L BICEP	
CHEST	
WAIST	
HIPS	
R THIGH	
L THIGH	
CALF	

NOTES

....
....
....
....
....
....
....
....
....
....
....

Workout Log Book

Date ....

WEIGHT MON / TUE / WED / THU / FRI / SAT / SUN

MUSCLE GROUP HOW I FEEL 1 / 2 / 3 / 4 / 5 / 6

START TIME FINISH TIME

WATER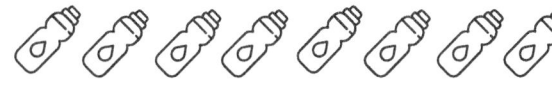

STRENGTH TRAINING

☐ UPPER BODY ☐ LOWER BODY ☐ ABS

CARDIO

EXERCISE	TIME	DISTANCE	CALS BURNED

EXERCISE	SET	1	2	3	4	5	6
	REPS						
	WEIGHT						
	REPS						
	WEIGHT						
	REPS						
	WEIGHT						
	REPS						
	WEIGHT						
	REPS						
	WEIGHT						
	REPS						
	WEIGHT						

EXERCISE	SET	1	2	3	4	5	6
	REPS						
	WEIGHT						
	REPS						
	WEIGHT						
	REPS						
	WEIGHT						
	REPS						
	WEIGHT						
	REPS						
	WEIGHT						
	REPS						
	WEIGHT						

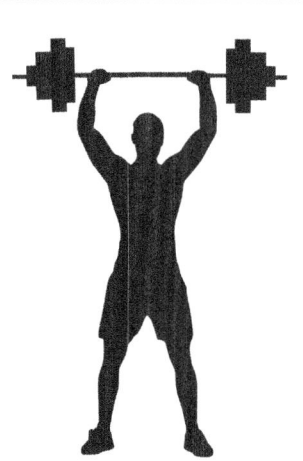

MEASUREMENTS	
NECK	
R BICEP	
L BICEP	
CHEST	
WAIST	
HIPS	
R THIGH	
L THIGH	
CALF	

NOTES

....
....
....
....
....
....
....
....
....
....
....

Workout Log Book

Date ....

WEIGHT MON / TUE / WED / THU / FRI / SAT / SUN

MUSCLE GROUP HOW I FEEL 1 / 2 / 3 / 4 / 5 / 6

START TIME FINISH TIME

WATER

STRENGTH TRAINING

☐ UPPER BODY ☐ LOWER BODY ☐ ABS

CARDIO

EXERCISE	TIME	DISTANCE	CALS BURNED

EXERCISE	SET	1	2	3	4	5	6
	REPS						
	WEIGHT						
	REPS						
	WEIGHT						
	REPS						
	WEIGHT						
	REPS						
	WEIGHT						
	REPS						
	WEIGHT						
	REPS						
	WEIGHT						

EXERCISE	SET	1	2	3	4	5	6
	REPS						
	WEIGHT						
	REPS						
	WEIGHT						
	REPS						
	WEIGHT						
	REPS						
	WEIGHT						
	REPS						
	WEIGHT						
	REPS						
	WEIGHT						

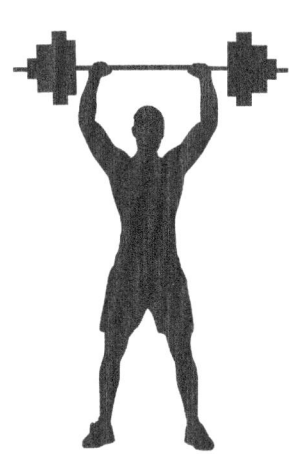

MEASUREMENTS	
NECK	
R BICEP	
L BICEP	
CHEST	
WAIST	
HIPS	
R THIGH	
L THIGH	
CALF	

NOTES

....
....
....
....
....
....
....
....
....
....
....

Workout Log Book

Date ....

WEIGHT MON / TUE / WED / THU / FRI / SAT / SUN

MUSCLE GROUP HOW I FEEL 1 / 2 / 3 / 4 / 5 / 6

START TIME FINISH TIME

WATER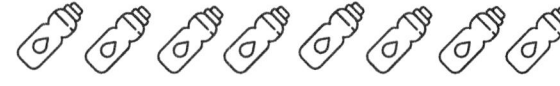

STRENGTH TRAINING

☐ UPPER BODY ☐ LOWER BODY ☐ ABS

CARDIO

EXERCISE	TIME	DISTANCE	CALS BURNED

EXERCISE	SET	1	2	3	4	5	6
	REPS						
	WEIGHT						
	REPS						
	WEIGHT						
	REPS						
	WEIGHT						
	REPS						
	WEIGHT						
	REPS						
	WEIGHT						
	REPS						
	WEIGHT						

EXERCISE	SET	1	2	3	4	5	6
	REPS						
	WEIGHT						
	REPS						
	WEIGHT						
	REPS						
	WEIGHT						
	REPS						
	WEIGHT						
	REPS						
	WEIGHT						
	REPS						
	WEIGHT						

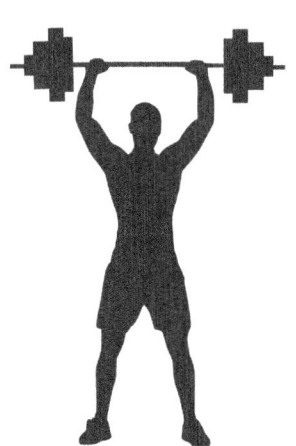

MEASUREMENTS	
NECK	
R BICEP	
L BICEP	
CHEST	
WAIST	
HIPS	
R THIGH	
L THIGH	
CALF	

NOTES

....
....
....
....
....
....
....
....
....
....
....

Workout Log Book

Date ....

WEIGHT MON / TUE / WED / THU / FRI / SAT / SUN

MUSCLE GROUP HOW I FEEL 1 / 2 / 3 / 4 / 5 / 6

START TIME FINISH TIME

WATER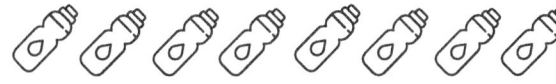

STRENGTH TRAINING

☐ UPPER BODY   ☐ LOWER BODY   ☐ ABS

CARDIO

EXERCISE	TIME	DISTANCE	CALS BURNED

EXERCISE	SET	1	2	3	4	5	6
	REPS						
	WEIGHT						
	REPS						
	WEIGHT						
	REPS						
	WEIGHT						
	REPS						
	WEIGHT						
	REPS						
	WEIGHT						
	REPS						
	WEIGHT						

EXERCISE	SET	1	2	3	4	5	6
	REPS						
	WEIGHT						
	REPS						
	WEIGHT						
	REPS						
	WEIGHT						
	REPS						
	WEIGHT						
	REPS						
	WEIGHT						
	REPS						
	WEIGHT						

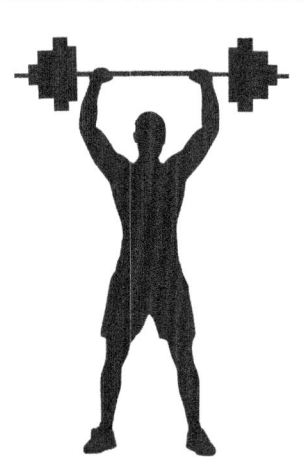

MEASUREMENTS	
NECK	
R BICEP	
L BICEP	
CHEST	
WAIST	
HIPS	
R THIGH	
L THIGH	
CALF	

NOTES

....
....
....
....
....
....
....
....
....
....
....
....

Workout Log Book

Date ....

WEIGHT MON / TUE / WED / THU / FRI / SAT / SUN

MUSCLE GROUP HOW I FEEL 1 / 2 / 3 / 4 / 5 / 6

START TIME FINISH TIME

WATER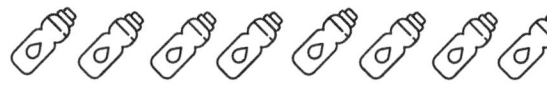

STRENGTH TRAINING

☐ UPPER BODY   ☐ LOWER BODY   ☐ ABS

CARDIO

EXERCISE	TIME	DISTANCE	CALS BURNED

EXERCISE	SET	1	2	3	4	5	6
	REPS						
	WEIGHT						
	REPS						
	WEIGHT						
	REPS						
	WEIGHT						
	REPS						
	WEIGHT						
	REPS						
	WEIGHT						
	REPS						
	WEIGHT						

EXERCISE	SET	1	2	3	4	5	6
	REPS						
	WEIGHT						
	REPS						
	WEIGHT						
	REPS						
	WEIGHT						
	REPS						
	WEIGHT						
	REPS						
	WEIGHT						
	REPS						
	WEIGHT						

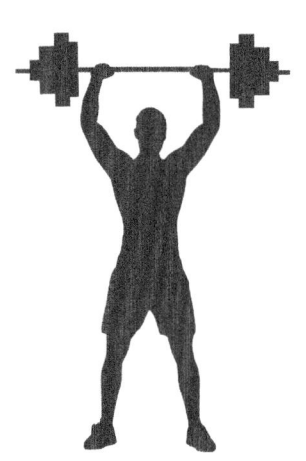

MEASUREMENTS	
NECK	
R BICEP	
L BICEP	
CHEST	
WAIST	
HIPS	
R THIGH	
L THIGH	
CALF	

NOTES

....
....
....
....
....
....
....
....
....
....
....

Workout Log Book

Date ....

WEIGHT MON / TUE / WED / THU / FRI / SAT / SUN

MUSCLE GROUP HOW I FEEL 1 / 2 / 3 / 4 / 5 / 6

START TIME FINISH TIME

WATER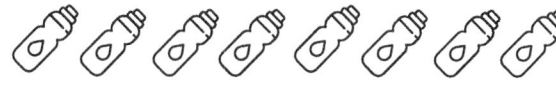

STRENGTH TRAINING

☐ UPPER BODY   ☐ LOWER BODY   ☐ ABS

CARDIO

EXERCISE	TIME	DISTANCE	CALS BURNED

EXERCISE	SET	1	2	3	4	5	6
	REPS						
	WEIGHT						
	REPS						
	WEIGHT						
	REPS						
	WEIGHT						
	REPS						
	WEIGHT						
	REPS						
	WEIGHT						
	REPS						
	WEIGHT						

EXERCISE	SET	1	2	3	4	5	6
	REPS						
	WEIGHT						
	REPS						
	WEIGHT						
	REPS						
	WEIGHT						
	REPS						
	WEIGHT						
	REPS						
	WEIGHT						
	REPS						
	WEIGHT						

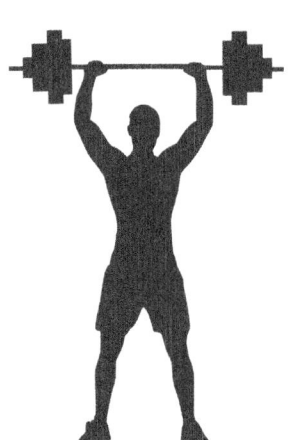

MEASUREMENTS	
NECK	
R BICEP	
L BICEP	
CHEST	
WAIST	
HIPS	
R THIGH	
L THIGH	
CALF	

NOTES

....
....
....
....
....
....
....
....
....
....
....

Workout Log Book

Date ....

WEIGHT MON / TUE / WED / THU / FRI / SAT / SUN

MUSCLE GROUP HOW I FEEL   1 / 2 / 3 / 4 / 5 / 6

START TIME FINISH TIME

WATER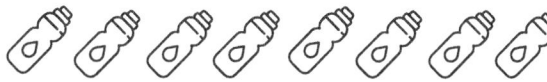

STRENGTH TRAINING

☐ UPPER BODY   ☐ LOWER BODY   ☐ ABS

CARDIO

EXERCISE	TIME	DISTANCE	CALS BURNED

EXERCISE	SET	1	2	3	4	5	6
	REPS						
	WEIGHT						
	REPS						
	WEIGHT						
	REPS						
	WEIGHT						
	REPS						
	WEIGHT						
	REPS						
	WEIGHT						
	REPS						
	WEIGHT						

EXERCISE	SET	1	2	3	4	5	6
	REPS						
	WEIGHT						
	REPS						
	WEIGHT						
	REPS						
	WEIGHT						
	REPS						
	WEIGHT						
	REPS						
	WEIGHT						
	REPS						
	WEIGHT						

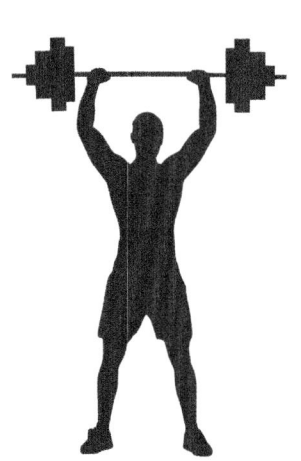

MEASUREMENTS	
NECK	
R BICEP	
L BICEP	
CHEST	
WAIST	
HIPS	
R THIGH	
L THIGH	
CALF	

NOTES

....
....
....
....
....
....
....
....
....
....
....

Printed in Great Britain
by Amazon